Creative Activities
For Health and Social Care

Maria Eales

ISBN:
ISBN-13: 978-1481811903
ISBN-10: 1481811908

DEDICATION

To my husband Mark, who is my greatest inspiration. The constant reminder of the cruelty of illness cannot and will not ever shield my eyes from the man that I married. He still stands in front of me today, a little more battered and in need of a stitch and a tartan patch over his threadbare bits but my man, nonetheless.

CONTENTS

INTRODUCTION

This book has been written specifically for the Edexcel specification of the First Diploma in Health and Social Care Unit 12 Creative and Therapeutic Activities. It contains all the underpinning knowledge, teaching activities and assignment brief for the unit.

Teachers can use this book to support classroom learning or students can use it as an independent learning resource.

Whilst theory is important for this unit, the kinesthetic learner can benefit from the practical elements and every effort should be made to allow students to explore as many creative activities as possible. This will equip them to plan and implement an appropriate activity for their work placement.

The cost of delivering this unit should not be underestimated and a range of resources will need to be made available to the student. Art and craft materials, a computer, a colour printer, board games, sporting equipment, a CD player, a working kitchen and a camera are the types of things that will be needed if students are to explore all the different types of activities in this unit.

Topic A.1 Different creative and therapeutic activities used in health and social care

We all have things that we *like* to do rather than things we *have* to do. Think about the types of things you do in the evening after work, school or college. You might like to play sport, *chill out* with your iPod, surf the Internet, go to a club or simply meet with friends and enjoy a hobby.

These kinds of activities make us feel happy but they are also important is many other ways. We learn new skills and remain physically and mentally active. We also maintain our sense of independence by making choices of the activities we undertake. We might make new friends or become more physically active.

Service users in health and social care organizations are no different and they need to be allowed to choose activities that they enjoy.

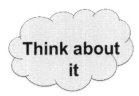

Think about it

Imagine a day when the only things you did were things that you had to do e.g., get dressed, eat meals, go to the toilet and go to bed. At all other times, you can either, sit in a chair and look out of the window or watch a television programme that doesn't interest you.

How would you feel?

What would you do?

Why is this situation wrong?

CARE SETTINGS

When we talk about care settings, we mean any kind of organization that provides a caring, supportive or educational service. These organisations may deal with specific age groups such as children, teenagers, adults or the elderly or they may be open to everyone.

A school, for example has pupils of a specific age group but a hospital is open to everyone, no matter what age they are. It is important that you are familiar with the different types of care settings in your area. You need to know who they provide a service for and the types of creative activities they organize.

Pre School, nursery provision and registered child minders.

These services provides care and educational services for children under 5 years old. Some pre schools are attached to primary schools. Children who attend these pre schools often have an easier time settling into full time school because they are already used to the school environment. All providers who care for children aged 3-5 years of age have to deliver the early years foundation stage curriculum. This is a set of criteria, set out by the Department of Education that helps children to learn new skills and develop healthily. Creative activities are central to this stage of development and learning is often encouraged through play and exploration of the world around them.

Residential and Nursing Care Homes.

A care home is a residential setting where a number of older people live, usually in single rooms, and have access to on-site care services. A home registered simply as a care home will provide personal care only - help with washing, dressing and giving medication. Some care homes are registered to meet a specific care need, for example dementia or terminal illness. Homes registered for nursing care may accept people who just have personal care needs but who may need nursing care in the future.

All care homes have to provide a programme of creative activities and this provision is monitored by inspectors from the Care Quality Commission.

Special Needs Schools

These schools are specifically designed to provide care and education services for children and young adults who have learning disabilities. All the teachers have specialist qualifications to assist the students learn at the rate they are able. Some schools are residential and students live there during term time. Others are day schools and operate like normal state schools.

Supported Living

This is a service that allows people with a disability to live independently in their own home or in a house with other disabled people. The care workers are there to offer whatever support is needed to allow the clients to live normal lives and make choices for themselves. This might mean that the care worker reminds the client where they have to go to take their library books back or how to pay money into their bank account. A shared house might have a programme of activities agreed by the residents. Friday nights might be DVD and a take away evening. Saturday morning might be a time when everyone goes swimming. The main concept of this type of living is that the residents have choices of what they do and don't want to do.

ACTIVITY 1

TYPES OF CARE SETTINGS

Complete the grid below by finding services in your local area and saying what they do and the age group they care for.

Setting	Age Group	Name of service	Types of creative activities?
Pre-School			
Residential care home			
Domiciliary Care Agency			
Special Needs School			
Supported living			

THE NEEDS OF THE INDIVIDUAL

All of us have needs and they can be split into four main areas:

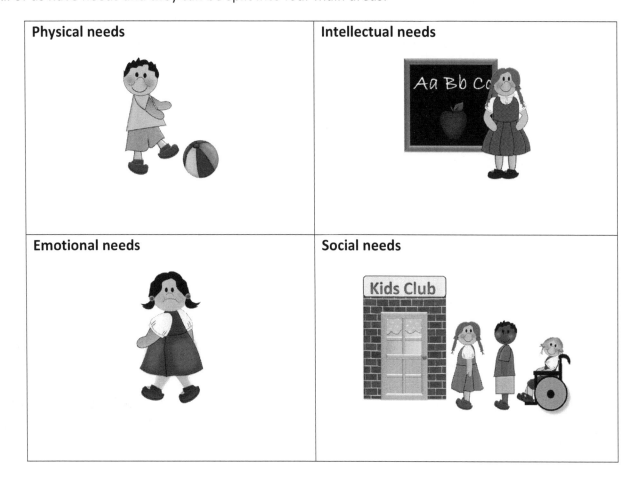

PHYSICAL NEEDS

All of us need to move around because if we don't, our muscles degenerate and our joints become stiff. Exercise is also very good for our body and if we increase our heart rate on a regular basis, it can decrease blood pressure and help to stop depression. From the day we are born we begin to develop fine and gross motor skills that we practice and maintain throughout our lives.

INTELLECTUAL NEEDS

Everyone needs to be able to think, learn new things, feel challenged, solve problems and recall memories. Human beings enjoy recalling and talking about things that have happened to them in the past. This is important because it reminds them of who they are, relationships they have formed with family members and friends.

Learning new things gives us all a sense of achievement. We feel a sense of success when we learn a new skill or solve a problem. Some people enjoy solving problems for fun, such as completing word puzzles or Sudoku games.

EMOTIONAL NEEDS

We all need a cuddle sometimes and this helps us when we are feeling emotionally low. Help and support from those people around us helps us to deal with emotional problems. It is also important for us to be able to express our emotions in an appropriate way. If a service user is feeling angry or frustrated about something, they should be given the opportunity to express their feelings without fear of rebuke.

Drama therapy is often used to allow people to display emotion in a safe environment. For example, an individual can write a short play that allows them to show anger about something in their life and then deal with it through the script.

In a similar way, if a service user is happy about something, like the birth of a grandchild, they should be allowed to share their joy and not be ignored.

SOCIAL NEEDS

The human being is a very social animal. We tend to like the company of others and we often become frightened and lonely when we do not have company. Everyone likes to have friends and family around them but we also need to have 'our own space' for when we want to be alone.

Service users in a care home have the right to entertain their family and friends in a private space, just like they would in their own home. Some care homes will put on a special 'birthday tea' for the client and invite their friends and family.

ACTIVITY 2

Read the section on the needs of the individual and the fill in the blank spaces to make correct sentences.

If we stop doing physical activities, our muscles _____ and our _____ become stiff. Doing

exercise that pushes our _____ rate up can reduce _____ _____ and help

to prevent _____.

Humans like the company of other _____ but they also like to have their _____

_____ for if they want to be alone.

Drama therapy allows people to show their _____ in an appropriate way. People should always

be _____ to show their _____ in a safe environment.

Language and communication is a part of our _____ . Deaf people may communicate using

_____ language. People who have had a stroke might point to pictures, words or symbols on

_____ _____.

Problem solving activities and puzzles can help to meet our _____ needs.

Missing Words

Own   Communication   Degenerate Emotions   Joints   Space   Allowed Heart Blood   Board
Culture Intellectual Display Pressure Feelings Sign Depression.

SUGGESTIONS FOR ACTIVITIES

Sports	Arts and Crafts	Music and Dancing
Golf	Card Making	Listening to music
Football	Knitting	Playing an instrument
Volley Ball	Sewing	Dance classes
Badminton	Painting	Singing
Swimming	Cooking	Drama groups
Gardening	**Walking or Travelling**	**Genealogy and History**
Planting	Guided walks	Researching family tree
Pruning	Treasure trails	Researching local history
Making tubs of plants	Visiting heritage sites	
	Visiting theme parks	
Games and Quizzes	**Reading, Writing and Storytelling**	**Photography**
Crosswords	Writing stories	Using photographs to make a scrapbook
Pub Quiz	Telling stories	Taking photographs
Chess	Community newsletter production	
Draughts	Visiting the library	
Card Games	Joining a book club	

ACTIVITY 3

Look at the table above that gives a range of different activities. Consider the different needs that can be met for each one. Write a P, I, L, E or S next to each activity. Physical, Intellectual, Language, Emotional or Social. Some activities might have more than one letter at the side of them.

MULTI SENSORY STIMULATION.

Multi-sensory stimulation uses all the senses of sight, hearing, touch, taste and smell to try and help a person's mental health and to help them understand their environment.

It's really useful for people with learning disabilities, sensory impairments and dementia. Many people with these types of conditions can become aggressive and this is usually linked to boredom and frustration. Multi sensory stimulation can be used to help relax a client and stimulate positive emotions like happiness.

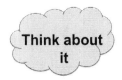

Imagine that you are deaf and blind. Which senses are you left with? How can these senses be used to stimulate you and help you make sense of the world around you?

Touch can be used to help you get around your environment. Sometimes, corridors in care homes have textured handrails to provide information on where the client is in the home. For example, bobbly handrails might mean that they are close to the lounge, whilst smooth handrails might be put close to bathrooms.

Smell can also be used to get around the care home. A lavender air freshener can mean the client is in the lounge and a rose air freshener might indicate that they are in their own bedroom.

Many people who lose one or more senses develop enhanced abilities in the other senses. So a blind person may be able to hear more things than they could before they lost their sight.

A texture book can be used to tell a story for a person with severe learning difficulties. Pages can have fur, silk, wool, sandpaper etc. stuck into their pages. The client can feel what a dog is like rather than being able to see or hear it.

Music is also a wonderful stimulus to invoke memories in the elderly. Playing appropriate music from years ago and talking to them about what they remember is a great way to get to know them and help them to remember their past.

ARTS THERAPY

Arts therapies are a way of using different arts such as, music, painting, dance, voice or drama to express your feelings and emotions.

You do not need any previous experience of the arts in order to participate in these activities. The main aim is to understand yourself better and discover your capabilities to deal with certain aspects of your life.

THERAPY PETS

Many people have pets at home and the love that they bring makes their owners feel happy and relaxed. School classroom often have small caged pets to teach the children how to care for an animal. Residential care homes often have a cat or a bird who bring great joy to the residents. Some residents. If they are able, can take responsibility for feeding the pet.

ACTIVITY 4

Have a look at the following websites and produce a power point presentation to show how animals are used to help ill or disabled people.

http://www.petsastherapy.org

http://www.animaltherapy.net

http://www.rda.org.uk

TOPIC A.2 THE BENEFITS OF CREATIVE AND THERAPEUTIC ACTIVITIES

PHYSICAL BENEFITS

Physical actions can be split into two areas; fine motor skills and gross motor skills.

Fine motor skills are the small but precise movements that we use to perform certain tasks. For example, we use our thumb and forefinger to hold a pen and form letters or draws shapes. This is a fine motor skill. We also use small, precise movements when we dial a number on our phone or type a word onto our computer keyboard.

A very young child has to learn these skills so when they first begin to draw, it appears just like scribbles on a piece of paper but as the practice, they develop the skills to draw a simple circle, a straight line and eventually a square. From this point they can learn to form letters by joining up dots. They can copy simple words that have been written for them and eventually, they learn to write letters, words and sentences in neat handwriting. These precise movement develops and improves hand eye co-ordination.

Cutting out shapes or cutting in a straight line is also a fine motor skill that has to be developed throughout childhood. Children have to learn about the dangers of using sharp cutting tools and they always need to be supervised very closely whilst they are using scissors.

The level of fine motor skills that a person has is often referred to as their *dexterity* and these skills need to be maintained and practiced regularly or it is easy for the individual to lose the skills. Throughout adulthood these skills are used on a daily basis from peeling vegetables to sewing a button on a shirt. Unfortunately, when we get to the elderly stage of our lives we often develop such things as arthritis in our hands that make it painful to perform these small movements. However, it is still important for the individual to continue to move around and perform tasks that are precise and intricate for as long as possible.

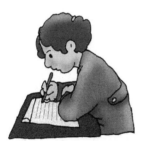 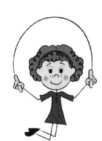 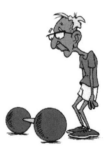

Gross motor skills involve bigger movements like walking, running, balancing and standing on tip toes. The human body is designed to move around quite a lot. It is not designed to sit on the couch eating crisps. By moving around we improve our muscle strength, bone density and we keep our joints mobile. Another advantage of vigorous exercise is the maintenance of a healthy cardio vascular system. Regular aerobic exercise reduces high blood pressure and burns fat to keep the body from becoming overweight.

Some scientific research suggests that exercise releases endorphins into the body. Endorphins are a 'feel good' chemical that reduces depression and makes us feel happy. The symptoms of stress can also be reduced by physical activity.

INTELLECTUAL BENEFITS

Our intellectual (or cognitive) abilities need to be practiced if we are going to maintain them. For example, if we wanted to learn the words to a song, we might listen to it several times, right the words down and then sing along to the song until we had remembered it all. However, if we did listen to the song or sing the song for a number of years, we would soon forget the words and music.

It is often said that as we get older, we begin to lose our ability to learn new things. This is simply not true unless we have a degenerative brain condition such as Alzheimer's disease. The elderly can learn new skills and they can improve their memory. A simple game to improve someone's memory is to place a number of items on a table and ask them to look at the items for about thirty seconds. Then ask them to close their eyes and you remove one or two items. When they open their eyes, they have to name the items that are no longer on the table. Obviously, the more items that are on the table, the more difficult the game is.

Problem solving is not just a skill that we use in everyday life but we also use it for fun. Doing word or math puzzles keeps our mind healthy and active.

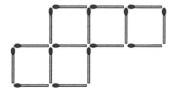

Move two matches to make four equal squares.

(Find the solution at the end of this book)

Puzzles can be completed alone or in a team. Teamwork encourages individuals to develop social skills as well as intellectual skills and can create a fun environment full of laughter and chatter. This improves communication with others and helps us to develop a broader vocabulary or practice words that we have already learnt. Social communication is important for a child's initial intellectual development and to sustain the communication skills that have been learnt.

A great deal of our communication is by body language and facial expressions. A child has to learn what these expressions mean and they learn these through social communication. A simple game of charades could be used to show children how we communicate with our bodies but the same game could also be used with an adult group to promote fun and emotional well being.

You have to measure exactly 4 liters of water, but you only have a 3-liter bottle and a 5-liter bottle. How do you do it?

EMOTIONAL BENEFITS

Our emotions are affected by our surroundings, our activities, our physical health and by people around us. Creative and therapeutic activities can help to improve our emotional well being by giving us a sense of achievement, a confidence boost or simply by making us laugh.

Boredom is an emotion that can be relieved by engaging in an activity. Sitting doing nothing is a recipe for depression and low self esteem. If we don't participate in activities, events, social communication, we will feel isolated and sad.

Producing something, such as a craft project or completing a puzzle gives us a sense of achievement and pride. We feel that we have succeeded in doing something and this makes us feel more confident about ourselves.

Our self esteem is the term we use to describe how we view oneself. A person with a high self esteem views themselves in positive light. It doesn't mean that they are being big headed, it just means that they can describe themselves using positive word. They recognize their own achievements and capabilities and this view is reinforced every time they do something and succeed.

On the other hand, an individual with a low self esteem will see themselves in a negative way. They might feel that they are a failure or incapable of doing anything right. It is hard to reverse this thought process but one of the ways it can be done is by using therapeutic activities to 'prove' to the individual that they are capable of achieving things.

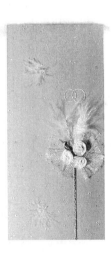

This card was made by a service user who attended a drop in center for people with mental health issues. She had been invited to a birthday party and she wanted to make a card to take with her.

She was very happy with the end result and even happier when the recipient showed everyone in the room because she was so impressed with the handiwork.

The service user had never made cards before but with the help of the activities coordinator at the center, she developed her skills and is now making cards to sell for charity. Now she describes herself as a craft worker rather than a person with a mental health problem, as she did before.

A retired math's teacher who was blind used to thrill and amaze care workers and other residents of the care home by doing complicated mental arithmetic problems that were asked of her. Cook regularly used to come and ask her to work out ratios for ingredients in recipes that she wanted to try out and children who visited the home used to try and pose number problems for him that he could not answer. He proved that he would still do addition more quickly that a calculator on his 86th birthday.

He had maintained his skills by practicing doing mental arithmetic every day since he retired. It was part of who he was and he didn't want to lose the ability to solve math problems because it was something that he enjoyed. It was essential for his emotional well being.

SOCIAL BENEFITS

Human beings are social animals. We like to communicate, laugh together, cry together, exchange views and ideas. Engaging in creative and therapeutic activities allow people to communicate with others who share their enjoyment.

Residents, staff and their families organized their own summer BBQ. Some of the residents were involved in preparing salads and side dishes. Others made the invitations and some participated by making decorations and flower displays for the dinning room. The gardening group at the home made sure that the hanging baskets and tubs were all looking their best and other residents chose the music that they wanted to play at the party.

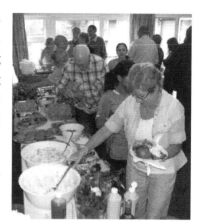

A budget committee was set up and they decided on how much they wanted to spend on the party and how much they would sell tickets for.

This community project was a great success and allowed people who had different skills to be involved at a level they could manage.

On a Wednesday afternoon at the home for young disabled adults, there is a music group. Some of the residents get together to play musical instruments or play music that they have heard on the radio or internet. It is a time for everyone to share their views about the latest pop music or the strange words they have found in a song that was released in the 1970s.

LANGUAGE BENEFITS

Whilst we're on the subject of social communication, I feel that we cannot ignore the benefits to language development. We have already mentioned the fact that children develop language skills through social interaction but language development does not stop once we have learnt the language. Adults continue to add to their vocabulary and we may even learn a second or third language. Only by interacting with others can we practice the language that we speak and add words to our vocabulary.

Sometimes, people who speak English as a second language may be able to get together with others who speak their native language. Polish groups or Italian groups may form simply for the purpose of conversing in the individuals mother tongue.

Deaf people might communicate using sign language or they may point to pictures or symbols using a communication board.

ACTIVITY 5

Using the grid below, make a list of the different types of activities that meets or benefits physical needs, intellectual needs, language needs, social needs and emotional needs.

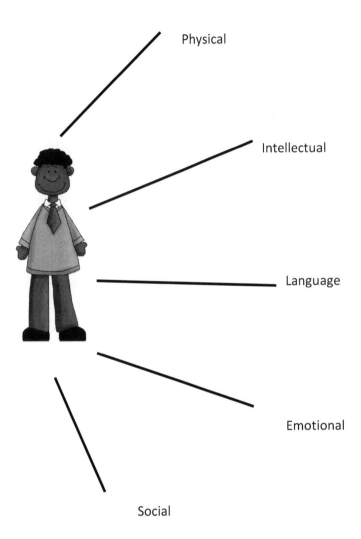

ACTIVITY 6

In pairs, brainstorm all the different things you can do or make with an empty jam jar can, a blank piece of A4 paper, a ball of string.

Item	Activities
An empty jam jar	
A blank piece of paper	
A ball of string	

Suggested Answers for Activity 6

Item	Activities
An empty jam jar	Make a holder for pens and pencils Paint it or cover it and make a flower vase Fill it will soil and grown cress.
A blank piece of paper	Origami Drawing and Painting Make a template for a sewing project
A ball of string	Macramé Weaving Gardening

CREATIVE ACTIVITIES AND GROUPS

Obviously, not everyone enjoys the same kinds of activities. A four year old might enjoy playing with a toy train but it is unlikely that an eighty-year-old woman will enjoy the same thing. Different groups enjoy different things and so we must consider a wide range of activities when thinking about service users needs in different care settings.

ACTIVITY 7

In small groups come up with some ideas for appropriate activities for service users in the following care settings. Remember to think of activities that meet physical, intellectual, language, emotional and social needs.

- A nursery
- A paediatric ward in a hospital
- A day centre for the over 65 age group.
- A residential care home for physically disabled young adults
- A school for young people with learning disabilities
- A prison
- A residential care home for the elderly

Now compare your results with other groups. Are your ideas different? Which activities appear to be the most common for each care setting?

STEREOTYPING

Stereotyping is making assumptions about a person or group of people based on their age, sex, culture, religion, health status or nationality. So when we are planning activities for service users we must be careful not to assume that people will like the activities that we think are appropriate. For example, not all older people like gardening and not all teenagers like rap music. It is vitally important that services users are given as many choices of activities, as possible.

RESOURCES

Unfortunately, when planning activities, we must consider the resources we have available. All organisations have a budget that can be spent on creative activities but it is usually small and so fund raising s often undertaken to pay for materials and equipment that are needed. In addition to this staffing has to be considered. Care organisations don't always have staff available to help with activities and so volunteers become a valuable resource. Often, activity organisers' have to become resourceful and collect recycled materials to use in activities. For example, the bottoms cut from empty 2 liter juice bottles can be made into plant pots. Old clothes can be cut up to provide fabric for needlecrafts. You must consider these things when planning your activities.

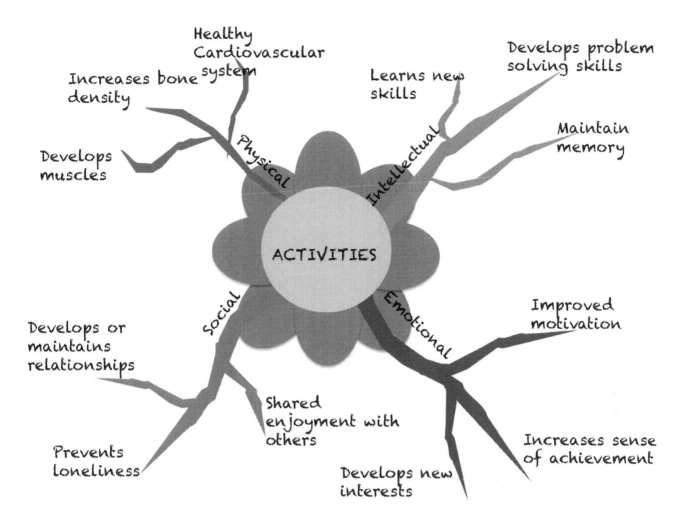

ACTIVITIY 8

The diagram above illustrates just some of the benefits of creative activities for the service user. There are many more. Can you design a display for your classroom or workroom to show a full range of benefits for clients?

ACTIVITY 9

Creative and therapeutic activities are beneficial for many different reasons. Can you think of some of them?

Physical Benefits

Intellectual Benefits

Social Benefits

Language Benefits

Emotional Benefits

Suggested answers for Activity 9

Physical Benefits

Helps us to stay physically active

Develops fine and gross motor skills

Promotes independence

Intellectual Benefits

Helps us to develop problem solving strategies

Gives us a sense of achievement (of winning) when we complete a puzzle or win a game

Helps us to improve our memory skills

Social Benefits

Helps us to make new friends or enjoy the company of existing ones.

Builds self esteem and prevents us from feeling lonely

Language Benefits

Increases vocabulary skills

Allows us to communicate in a way that we find comfortable

Emotional Benefits

Promotes happiness and lessens feelings of isolation

Improves self esteem.

LET'S EXPLORE A CREATIVE ACTIVITY

Below you will see an activity plan for a group of people who are recovering after a stroke. They are various stages of recovery and so the gardening activity has been split into three levels to allow everyone to participate.

ACTIVITY PLAN: GARDENING AND CARE OF PLANTS

Define Social Group	A group of adults aged 48 to 76 who have suffered a stroke and are at varying stages of recovery
Aims of the activity	**Physical**: To improve mobility and develop fine and gross motor skills **Intellectual:** To encourage services users to share existing knowledge and learn new facts. **Language:** To encourage service users to communicate with other on a specific topic. **Emotional:** To promote enjoyable activities and increase happiness score of the service users. **Social:** To encourage services users to socialise with other who share their enjoyment of gardening.

LEVEL 1	LEVEL 2	LEVEL 3
Watering indoor plants with a watering can Pulling dead heads off plants Choosing plants or seeds from a catalogue Visiting a garden center Share their existing knowledge.	Planting seeds or young plants into small pots Using a trowel to transplant small plants into larger tubs Watering plants with a larger watering can Weeding a flower border Communicating with others about plants Share their existing knowledge	Putting compost into large tubs Transplanting larger plants or small trees Using a hosepipe to water outdoor plants Pruning bushes and shrubs Share their existing knowledge or new facts that have been learnt

Resources: Large and small watering cans, hosepipe, seedling plant pots, seed catalogues, packets of seeds or small plants, small trowel, flower tubs, potting compost, larger plants or trees, pruning sheers, gardening books or magazines.

Communication aids eg word cards, pictures.

Cost: Staffing cost for two hours, cost of materials. Estimated £100.00

ACTIVITY 10

Now it is your turn to plan an activity. Below you will find an activity plan that has only given you details of the activity and the social group. You must complete the rest of the planning sheet.

ACTIVITY PLAN: SEWING A FELT DECORATION		
Define Social Group	A group of six young adults aged 13 to 16 who have learning difficulties.	
Aims of the activity	**Physical**: **Intellectual**: **Language**: **Emotional**: **Social**:	
LEVEL 1	**LEVEL 2**	**LEVEL 3**
Resources:		
Communication aids		
Cost:		

ACTIVITY 11 LET'S DO AN ACTIVITY

The following activity can be completed as either a sewing project or a paper craft project. You will see below, a pattern to make a cup cake decoration.

What you will need:

Three pieces of coloured felt or three pieces coloured of card

A pair of scissors

Sewing Thread or glue

A needle for a sewing project.

What you need to do

Print off the pattern for the cup cake on the next page.

Cut round the individual pieces and then cut round the edge of the full cupcake. Use the full cupcake as the backing and then sew or stick the individual pieces onto the front of the full cupcake.

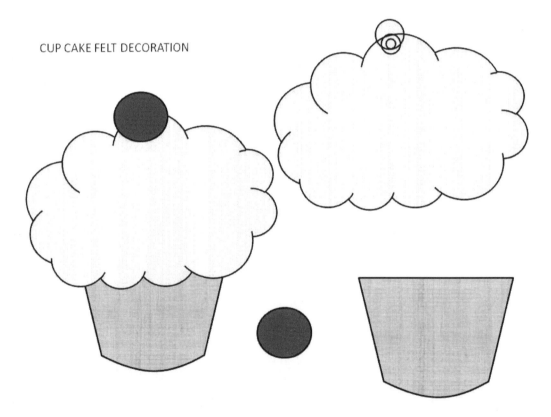

CUP CAKE FELT DECORATION

ACTIVITY 12

Once you have completed the cupcake activity, you will need to evaluate it to decide on how appropriate it is for specific client groups.

EVALUATION
Were there any things that you would change, now that you have completed the project?
Which social groups would it be appropriate for and which ones wouldn't it be appropriate for?
How much would this project cost for an individual service user and is this cost prohibitive?
What health and safety aspects must be taken into consideration when completing this project with service users?
Could this project be extended or simplified to meet the needs of more or less able service users?

TOPIC B.1 THE ROLE OF PROFESSIONALS IN HELPING AND ENCOURAGING INDIVIDUALS.

There are a range of professionals who help and encourage individuals to take part in creative and therapeutic activities.

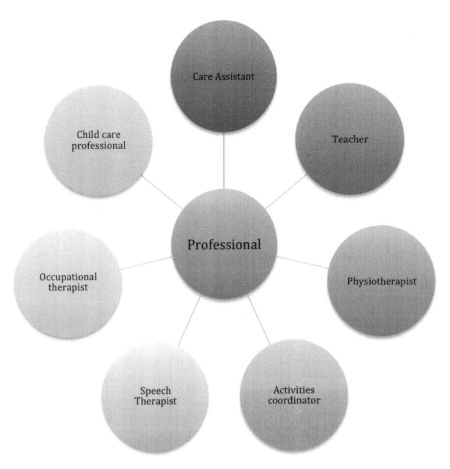

ACTIVITY 13

In groups of four, brain storm ideas about the kind of things these professionals might do to help their clients to participate in activities.

WAYS PROFESSIONAL SUPPORT ACTIVITIES

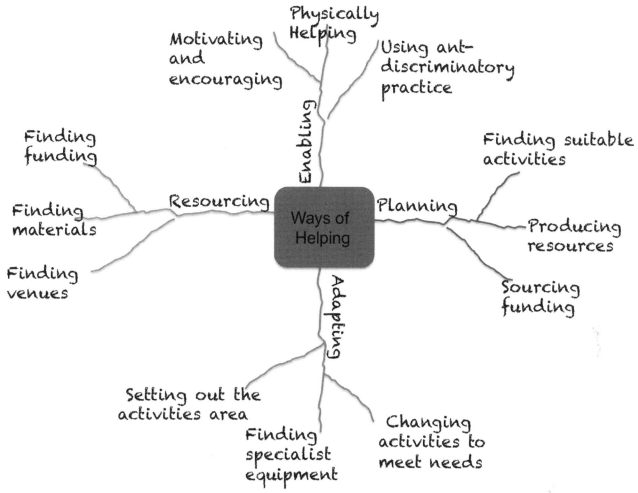

Anyone who is planning an activity needs to put a lot of thought into the planning stage. The first thing that needs to be done is suitable activities must be chosen. These must be age and capability appropriate. It's no use organizing a skiing trip for a group of elderly disabled people, it would be just plain dangerous! A better idea might be a applique sewing activity. This may involve the activity organizer cutting out the shapes for the clients to sew onto the backing material.

Finding and raising funding is a large part of an activity organizer's job. Most organizations have a small budget for activities but it is seldom enough to give a full range of choice. Usually the activities organizer must either apply for funding from various agencies or by raising money themselves.

ORGANISATIONS THAT CAN PROVIDE FUNDING

The Arts Council http://www.artscouncil.org.uk

Farming and Countryside Education http://www.face-online.org.uk

Awards for All http://www.awardsforall.org.uk/england/index.html

Volunteers are an important resource when organizing activities. Have a look at the following case study.

Alice The Volunteer.

I have been a volunteer at Sunnyside Residential Care home for five years and I am responsible for organizing creative activities for the twenty residents. The yearly budget for all activities is only £150 so I have to do a lot of begging and borrowing to make sure that activities go ahead.

Four times a year, I organize a *'bring and buy'* sale or a craft sale to raise money for a coach trip to the seaside. I have to enlist the help of other volunteers and off duty staff to push the residents' wheelchairs when we get there. Last year we raised £572 and it allowed us to go on a day trip and buy plants for our garden. We also used some of the money to buy materials for the craft room. We like to make cards to sell and we also make dried flower arrangements.

One of the residents is interested in photography and he takes photographs of our events and we make a display in the entrance hall. Two of the ladies like to knit and we ask relatives and friends to bring in any wool they might have left over from their own crafts. Last year, we bought a new CD player and we borrow CDs from the Library so that we can all have a good sing song.

We do have some residents who like to become involved in food preparation and they often volunteer to prepare vegetables for lunch. We even have one lady who likes to bake a cake occasionally. We have to help her to weigh out the ingredients and work the automatic mixer but she loves to offer the cake around at tea time.

ACTIVITY 14

List the activities that are undertaken by the residents in this care home.

Explain the kind of fund raising activities that help to fund the activities

What kind of equipment would be needed for the activities to take place?

Can you suggest any other activities that might be appropriate for the residents?

ACTIVITY 15

Alan is 85 years old. He has spent all his life living in England and he used to love to dance with his wife when they were in his twenties. He also recalled that, when he was a little boy, his mother and father used to dance to something called 'swing'.

1. What year was Alan born?
2. Which decade would he have been in his twenties?
3. Make a list of ten popular songs that Alan may have danced to with his wife
4. Make a list of five songs that he may have watched his mother and father dance to.
5. Explain why memories are important.

ACTIVITY 16

Have a look at the chart below and then fill in the column at the side of each professional to say how they might support activities. You may need to do some research to find the answers.

Professional	What do they do to make activities possible?
Teacher	
Health Care Assistant	
Prison Officer	
Occupational Therapist	
Speech Therapist	
Social Care Assistant	

ETHICAL CONSIDERATONS WHEN PLANNING ACTVITIES

It isn't acceptable to simply organize an activity without consulting the service users. They are entitled to choose what they like to do. It is also unacceptable to force someone to join in when they don't want to. An individual's needs must also be taken into consideration when planning activities.

ANTI DISCRIMINATORY PRACTICE

Anyone who organizes an activity must bear in mind the participants right to be allowed to join in regardless of their spiritual beliefs, culture, language, disability, race, lifestyle choices, sexual orientation or gender preferences. This sometimes means that an activity may have to be adapted to meet an individual's personal needs.

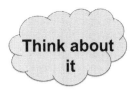

Taking a group of elderly people on a long coach trip might cause problems with continence issues. What other problems need to be taken into consideration when you know that you have got a diabetic person, a person with arthritis in their hips and knees and a vegetarian?

Organizing a Christmas party for a group of multi ethnic young adults. You have five Christian people, two Jewish people, one agnostic person and one person who doesn't like parties. What could you do to make sure everyone has an opportunity to be involved?

Taking a group of disabled adults swimming might cause problems in the changing rooms. What could you do to make sure they are treated with respect and ensure their dignity?

ACTIVITY 17

Imagine you are working in a special needs school and you have three Jewish pupils, five catholic pupils and six that follow no particular religion. You want to put on a special lunch for students, friends and family. You want all the students to be involved in preparing the food.

Make a list of the type of food that would be suitable to meet the needs of everyone's spiritual beliefs.

Make a list of things that you will need to consider when organizing the kitchen to allow the students to prepare the food.

TOPIC C.1 PLAN AND IMPLEMENT APPROPRIATE ACTIVITIES

HEALTH AND SAFETY

This is a very important aspect of planning activities and there are laws to protect both services users and staff. These laws must be adhered to during the planning, implementation and tidying up after activities.

The Health and Safety at Work Act 1974

This is the main piece of legislation for keeping people safe. It doesn't just cover employees but also applies to service users, visitors to the organization and anyone else who is involved in the activities. This Act requires that the organization assesses the risks involved with any activity and puts procedures in place to protect everyone.

The activities must take place in an area that has appropriate ventilation, temperature and lighting. There must be access to toilet and hand washing facilities. All equipment must be checked regularly to make sure they are working properly and are safe.

The area must be kept safe at all times, so things shouldn't be left on the floor in case someone trips over them. Any spills must be cleaned up immediately and any hazardous chemical must be disposed of correctly.

Correct protective clothing must be worn if it needed for either assisting in activities or performing activities. If a service user needs help with moving and handling, correct techniques must be used by suitably qualified staff. This means that they must have completed a moving and handling course and they must use the appropriate equipment.

Reporting of Injuries, Diseases and Dangerous Occurrences Regulations 1995 (RIDDOR)

Employers, the self-employed and those in control of premises are required by law to report specified workplace incidents, such as work-related deaths, major injuries, 7-day injuries (those causing more than seven day's inability to carry out normal duties), work related diseases, and dangerous occurrences (near miss accidents). They are also required to report an accident to the general public where the person has been taken to hospital. AN accident book must be kept on the premises and all accidents must be documented in the book. The records must be accurate, up to date and completed by witnesses and injured persons.

The Control of Substances Hazardous to Health Regulations 2002 (COSHH)

This piece of legislation relates to the storage and disposal of any type of waste that is hazardous to health. For example, if you take an incontinent person on a day trip, you must make arrangements for the safe disposal of their incontinence pad or soiled clothing. If you are using paint or paint cleaning materials, they must be disposed of appropriately and not poured down the kitchen sink. All substances that may be hazardous to health have to be stored correctly and kept away from vulnerable people, such as children or those with dementia.

RISK ASSESSMENTS

Risks are part of everyday life. We all face risks from the moment we get up to the moment we go to sleep. In fact, we are even at risk whilst we are asleep....we could fall out of bed and injure ourselves.

The law does not expect organisations to completely eliminate risk but it does expect them to complete a risk assessment and put measures in place people as is reasonably possible.

The first thing that needs to be done is to identify the *hazard.* A hazard is something that has the potential to cause harm. A risk is the level of likelihood that the hazard will cause harm. This is often judged as low medium and high

So let's have a look at an example and assess the risk.

Hazard	Situation	Level of Risk
Strong Glue	Adults who are mentally and physically fit and understand the correct way to use the glue.	Low
Strong Glue	Children with learning difficulties who like to put things in their mouth.	High
Strong Glue	Elderly residents of a care home who understand how to use the glue but sometimes get a bit forgetful.	Medium

When planning activities, the organiser must look at several different types of hazard: Physical, environmental, chemical and emotional.

A physical hazard is something like a piece of equipment or furniture. An example of an environmental hazard could be the weather or the levels of ventilation in a room. A chemical hazard could be something like paint or glue. An emotional hazard might be putting people in a situation that causes them to become upset.

Remember that for each activity you plan, you will need to complete a risk assessment form and explain how you will manage the hazards and reduce the risks.

ACTIVITY 18

Let's assess the risks of some activity items for three different social groups. In the boxes under each group say if the risk for each piece of equipment is High, Medium or Low

Item	For Elderly Dementia	For Teenagers with Drug Problems	For children aged 5 and below
Sharp craft knife			
Hairdryer			
Balloons already blown up			
Paint brush			
Pen			

ACTIVITY 19: Card making – Let's try it out.

Target Audience: Ages adults. Group size 12 adults.

Aims of the activity: To produce a greetings card for ay of a birthday. To encourage social interaction between group members. To promote independent thought and choice.

Skills to be developed: Fine motor skills through cutting shapes from card. Language skills through discussing their ideas with other people. Intellectual skills through learning a new technique. Social skills though working with other people.

Resources you will need:

12 pairs of scissors

Templates for the toppers for the cards (see templates page)

24 sheets of A4 different coloured card

Glue and sticky pads

A computer and printer for printing pictures, words, backing papers etc.

A range of card crafting papers, ribbons toppers or magazines.

Instructions.

Each person should take a piece of neutral coloured A4 and fold it in half to make the blank card. Alternatively, you could use read made card blanks that are available quite cheaply from stationary shops or the Internet.

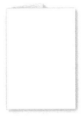

Now show the adults in the group pictures of different types of cards that can be produced. These can be found easily on the Internet.

Encourage people to discuss ideas for their own cards. Show them the materials that are available to them. Promote a friendly environment by chatting and use of appropriate humour.

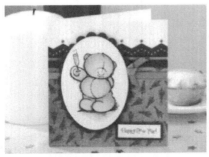
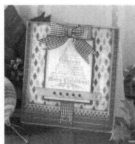
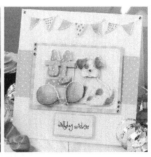

They key thing for this activity is to promote independence and avoid giving specific instructions, like you would with children.

You will need to practice making cards or research card making on the internet before you begin this activity with adults.

Notes

Raised sticky pads are pieces of foam that are sticky on either side. They are used to raise part of a picture up from the back ground picture to give a 3D effect.

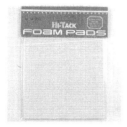

TEMPLATES FOR GREETINGS CARDS

NB: Remember that these are only ideas and, if possible, the service users should be encouraged to design their own.

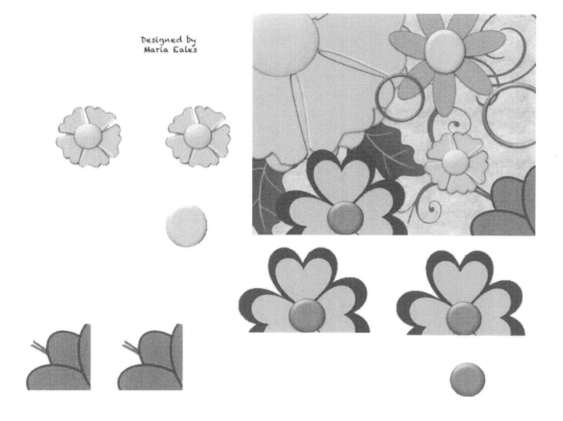

Each shape is cut out and stuck onto the original picture, using raised sticky pads. It can then be attached to the card.

ACTIVITY 20

Produce your own evaluation sheet and evaluate this activity for the target group. Remember to include costing for the activity and make recommendations for how it could be improved or completed more cheaply.

ACTIVITY 21: Name That Tune.

Target Audience: Teenagers and adults. Group size: above 6.

Aims of the activity: To engage adults in group activities where teams of people compete to name the title of a song.

Skills to be developed: Language skills through discussing their ideas with other people. Intellectual skills through making use of memory. Social skills though working with other people.

Resources you will need:

A tape recorder or CD player

A selection of age appropriate music

Quiz sheets

Answer sheet for the competition host

Pens to write down their answers

Instructions.

People should be encouraged to get into teams of two or more and be given a pen and an answer sheet.

You will play the beginning of a song and ask them to 'name that tune'. Depending on the group, you must judge how much of the song you play. I usually play the first verse of a song but not the part where it gives the title away. The teams then write their answers down on the ir answer sheet and you go onto the next song.

Remember that the songs need to be age appropriate so it's not use playing sounds from the 1960s to a group of teenagers.

ACTIVITY 22

Now it is your turn to plan, implement and evaluate an activity for the people in your class.

In groups of four, plan an activity that takes fifteen to thirty minutes for the members of your class. Remember that it must be age appropriate, affordable, uses resources that you have collected or recycled.

Once your classmates have completed your activity, you must hand them an evaluation sheet so that they can feedback to you on recommendations for improvements.

Solution to matchstick puzzle

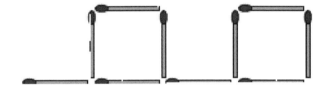

ASSIGNMENT BRIEF

GRADING CRITERIA

LEVEL 1 PASS	LEVEL 2 PASS	LEVEL 2 MERIT	LEVEL 2 DISTINCTION
A.1 Identify three creative and therapeutic activities suitable for individuals or groups in one health and social care setting.	2A.P1 Describe three creative and therapeutic activities suitable for individuals or groups in two different health and social care settings.		
1A.2 Outline the benefits of three creative and therapeutic activities for individuals or groups in one health and social care setting.	2A.P2 Describe the benefits of three creative and therapeutic activities for individuals or groups in two different health and socialsettings.	2A.M1 Assess the suitability of creative and therapeutic activities for an individual or group, with reference to a case study.	2A.D1 Make recommendations to improve creative and therapeutic activities for an individual or group, with reference to a case study.
1B.3 Outline the role of professionals who plan and implement activities in the health and social care setting	2B.P3 Describe the role of professionals when planning and implementing activities in one health and social care settings.	2B.M2 Compare and contrast the role of two professionals when planning and implementing activities in one health and social care settings.	2B.D2 Evaluate the impact of professional support on a selected individual participating in creative and therapeutic activities.
1C.4 Describe three factors that affect the selection, planning and implementation of creative and therapeutic activities.	2C.P4 Describe factors that affect the selection, planning and implementation of creative and therapeutic activities in one health and social care setting.		
1C.5 Plan one creative and therapeutic activity for service users of one health and social care setting.	2C.P5 Select, plan and implement, one individual or one group creative and therapeutic activity for service users in one health and social care setting.	2C.M3 Assess the selection, planning and implementation of the creative and therapeutic activity	2C.D3 Recommend improvements to the planning and implementation of the creative and therapeutic activity

TASK 1

Successful completion of this task will allow you to achieve grading criteria 1A.P1, 1A.P2, 2A.P1, 2A.P2.

A community center in your local town wants to provide activity days for a range of different social groups. They have asked you to provide a power point presentation on four different activities and the benefits to the service users.

TASK 2

Successful completion of this task will allow you to achieve grading criteria 2A. M1 and 2A.D1

A group of 10 children attend an after school club for an hour and a half, at their local community center. One of the children only has one hand and another of the children is partially blind. The activity coordinator has planned an activity for the children, which is baking some fairy cakes.

Assess the suitability of this activity for the group and then make recommendations as to how this activity could be improved to meet everyone's needs.

Think about things such as health and safety, special equipment, cost of resources, the needs of the group and the time factors involved.

TASK 3

Successful completion of this task will allow you to achieve grading criteria 1B.3, 2B.P3, 2B.M2 and 2B.D2

The staff at the community center are very pleased with your recommendations for the improvements of their cookery activity but they are unsure of what their roles will be.

Produce a grid or written report to explain how each member of staff can support and encourage the children to successfully participate in the group activity.

The staff are:

Activities Coordinator

A care Assistant

A Parent volunteer

Once you have done this, write a short paragraph to compare the roles of the staff members in terms of responsibilities evaluate the impact of professional support on a the disabled individuals participating in creative and therapeutic activities.

TASK 4

Successful completion of this task will allow you to achieve grading criteria 1C.4 and 2C.P4

Produce a diagram to describe at least three factors that affect the selection, planning and implementation of creative and therapeutic activities in one health and social care setting.

You might use a spider diagram to complete this task.

TASK 5

Successful completion of this task will allow you to achieve grading criteria 1C.4 and 2C.P4

The community center has asked you to take part in implementing some of their creative and therapeutic activities. They have asked you to plan one activity and submit the plans to them. You will also need to ensure that you are clear about how legislation, guidelines and Codes of Practice govern what they do.

You must then implement and evaluate your activity.

ABOUT THE AUTHOR

Maria Eales is an experienced and qualified teacher who has worked in schools and colleges across the UK. Her vibrant teaching style, coupled with her creative nature has lead her to a second career as a writer and producer of exciting teaching resources.

Printed in Great Britain
by Amazon.co.uk, Ltd.,
Marston Gate.